HEALTHY BARIATRIC JUICING AND SMOOTHIE RECIPES BOOK

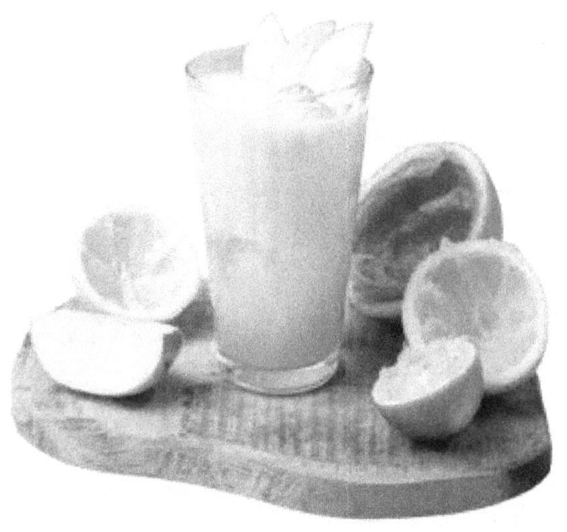

40 Nourishing, Tasty, and Easy Nutrient-Rich Blends for High-Protein Smoothies and Shakes

Dr. Linda B. Allen

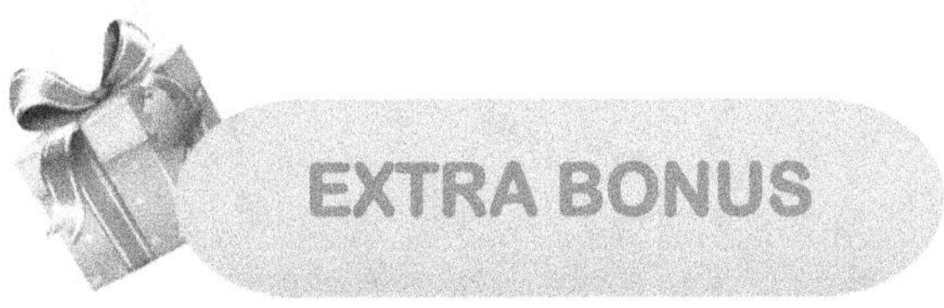

BONUS

12 EXERCISES FOR GASTRIC SLEEVE

BARIATRIC PATIENTS

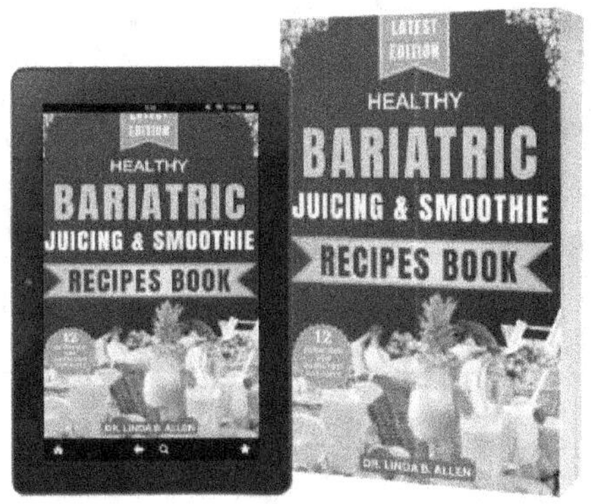

SCAN THE QR-CODE BELOW FOR MORE BOOKS FROM THIS AUTHOR

TABLE OF CONTENTS

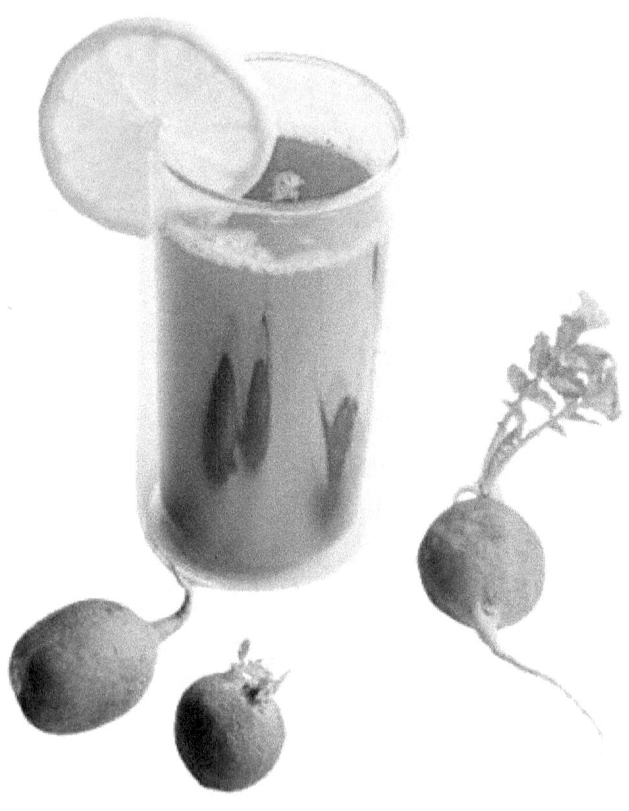

INTRODUCTION

I am Dr. Linda B. Allen, a passionate advocate for patient-centered care and a dedicated expert in the field of diet and nutrition. It is with great pleasure that I present to you my latest endeavor, a nutritional treasure trove crafted specifically for those who have undergone gastric sleeve bariatric surgery.

This project was born out of a deeply personal connection to the impact of bariatric procedures on individuals' lives. Inspired by the remarkable recovery of my own cousin sister, who, under my guidance, navigated her post-surgery days with resilience and embraced a healthier lifestyle, I am thrilled to share my expertise in a more focused realm: the realm of nourishing and rejuvenating smoothies and juices.

Before diving into the delectable world of nutrient-rich blends, it's essential to acknowledge the success of my previous cookbook, the ***"Gastric Sleeve Bariatric Cookbook for Beginners"*** Witnessing my cousin sister's swift and successful recovery.

Thanks to the wholesome recipes and strategic meal plans outlined in that book, fueled my commitment to further explore and refine nutritional support for bariatric patients.

Recognizing the unique dietary needs and challenges faced by gastric sleeve bariatric patients, I found a compelling need to delve into a more specific facet of nutrition, the world of rejuvenating smoothies and invigorating juices. These liquid marvels not only offer a refreshing departure from conventional meals but also present an efficient and enjoyable way to meet the heightened protein and nutrient requirements crucial for post-surgery recovery.

This brings us to my latest creation, "Healthy Bariatric Juicing and Smoothie Recipes Book: 40 Nourishing, Tasty, and Easy Nutrient-Rich Blends for High-Protein Smoothies and Shakes." Drawing upon my extensive medical background and hands-on experience in bariatric nutrition, this book is more than just a collection of recipes; it's a comprehensive guide to embracing a delicious and health-conscious lifestyle after gastric sleeve bariatric surgery.

Embark on this culinary and nutritional adventure with me, as we unlock the potential of bariatric juicing and smoothies, the perfect companions on your path to wellness after gastric sleeve bariatric surgery.

Understanding Bariatric Nutrition

The first step in navigating the world of bariatric nutrition is comprehending the unique dietary needs that follow surgical interventions. Bariatric surgery, such as the gastric sleeve procedure, alters the anatomy of the digestive system, necessitating a strategic approach to nutrition. It's not just about quantity but quality, ensuring that every nutrient counts towards optimal recovery and overall well-being.

One key aspect of bariatric nutrition is the prioritization of protein intake. Proteins play a crucial role in tissue repair, muscle maintenance, and immune function, essential elements for a swift and successful recovery. A bariatric diet rich in lean proteins ensures that the body receives the necessary building blocks for healing and sustained vitality.

Equally important is the focus on nutrient-dense foods. Post-surgery, the capacity for food intake may be reduced, emphasizing the importance of choosing foods that pack a nutritional punch.

Incorporating a variety of fruits, vegetables, whole grains, and lean proteins becomes paramount to address vitamin and mineral requirements.

Navigating portion control becomes an art in bariatric nutrition. Smaller, well-balanced meals not only aid digestion but also prevent overloading the system. It's not about deprivation but about crafting meals that maximize nutritional value within the constraints of the altered digestive capacity.

In essence, understanding bariatric nutrition is about creating a dietary landscape that supports healing, enhances energy levels, and fosters long-term health. It is a journey of informed choices, mindful eating, and a commitment to well-being.

Benefits of Juicing and Smoothies for Bariatric Patients:

Enter the world of juicing and smoothies, a delightful avenue to elevate the bariatric nutrition experience. Beyond being a refreshing treat for the taste buds, these liquid marvels offer a spectrum of benefits that align seamlessly with the unique needs of post-bariatric life.

First and foremost, juicing and smoothies provide a convenient and enjoyable way to meet heightened protein requirements. Blending together protein-rich ingredients, such as Greek yogurt, nut butters, or protein powder, results in delicious concoctions that effortlessly contribute to the daily protein goals crucial for recovery.

The texture of these beverages offers a gentle introduction to solid foods, making them particularly appealing during the initial stages of post-surgery dietary progression. They become a bridge between clear liquids and more substantial meals, aiding in the gradual adaptation of the digestive system.

The hydration factor cannot be overlooked. Bariatric patients are often encouraged to stay well-hydrated, and juicing and smoothies offer a dual advantage by providing both fluids and essential nutrients. This becomes especially important as proper hydration supports digestion, prevents constipation, and facilitates nutrient absorption.

Variety becomes the spice of life, and the same holds true for bariatric nutrition.

Juicing and smoothies open up a world of flavor combinations, allowing individuals to explore diverse tastes and textures. This not only enhances the culinary experience but also promotes adherence to a health-conscious lifestyle.

Moreover, the inherent versatility of these beverages accommodates the inclusion of a wide range of fruits, vegetables, and superfoods. This diversity ensures a broad spectrum of vitamins and minerals, contributing to the overall nutritional robustness of the bariatric diet.

In essence, juicing and smoothies emerge as nutritional allies, offering a pleasurable and practical means to elevate the bariatric nutrition experience. They transcend the realm of mere beverages, becoming a dynamic and flavorful component of the path to wellness.

Tools and Equipment for Successful Blending:

As we embark on the journey of incorporating juicing and smoothies into bariatric nutrition, the right tools and equipment become our trusty companions in this culinary adventure. These essential elements not only simplify the blending process but also enhance the overall experience, making it accessible and enjoyable for everyone.

High-Quality Blender: The Heart of the Operation

A reliable blender is the linchpin of successful blending. Opt for a high-quality blender with sufficient power to effortlessly process a variety of ingredients, including frozen fruits, vegetables, and ice. Investing in a blender with variable speeds and preset programs ensures versatility, allowing you to achieve the desired consistency for different recipes.

Nutrient Extraction Tools: Harnessing the Goodness

To maximize the nutritional yield of your blends, consider adding nutrient extraction tools to your arsenal. These may include a juicer for extracting liquid from fruits and vegetables, ensuring that every drop of goodness is captured. Nutrient extraction tools complement the blender, providing flexibility in crafting a diverse range of beverages.

Measuring Tools: Precision in Portions

Achieving the perfect balance of ingredients is key to crafting blends that are both delicious and nutritionally sound. Measuring cups, spoons, and kitchen scales become invaluable tools for precision in portion control.

This attention to detail ensures that each blend aligns with the recommended nutritional guidelines for post-bariatric life.

Storage Containers: Convenience and Portability

Anticipating the need for convenience and portability, invest in a selection of storage containers suitable for both preparation and on-the-go consumption. Mason jars, portable smoothie cups, and airtight containers make it easy to store pre-prepared ingredients and blended creations, facilitating a seamless integration of juicing and smoothies into daily life.

Educational Resources: Empowering Knowledge

Equip yourself with educational resources that demystify the art of blending and offer insights into the nutritional content of various ingredients. Books, online guides, and reputable websites become valuable companions, empowering you with the knowledge to make informed choices and experiment with creative recipes.

By assembling the right tools and equipment, you transform your kitchen into a vibrant workshop where ingredients are elevated to liquid gold. This not only streamlines the blending process but also paves the way for a culinary journey filled with exploration, innovation, and the joy of crafting nourishing beverages tailored to your bariatric needs.

Understanding bariatric nutrition is a voyage of self-discovery, where informed choices and mindful practices form the foundation of post-surgery well-being. Juicing and smoothies, with their myriad benefits, become not just beverages but vibrant expressions of a health-conscious lifestyle. Armed with the right tools and equipment, this journey unfolds as a delightful adventure, inviting you to savor the flavors of rejuvenation and embrace the boundless possibilities that bariatric nutrition has to offer.

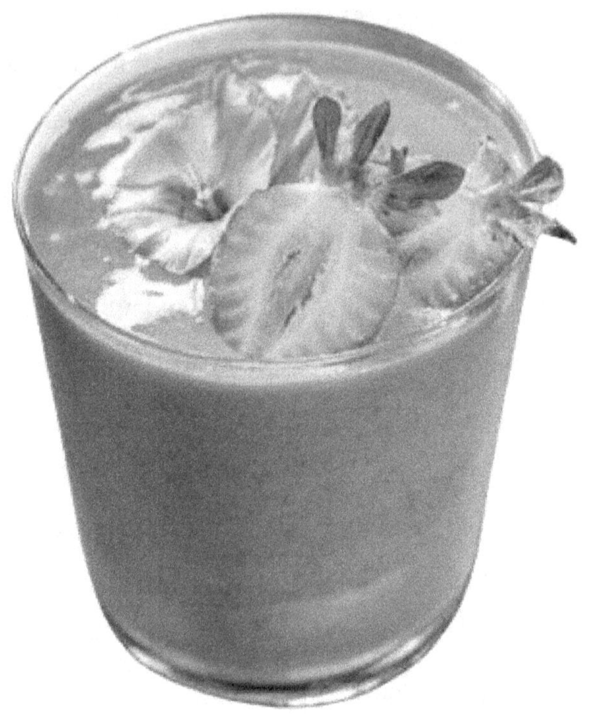

BUILDING BLOCKS OF NUTRIENT-RICH BLENDS

Embarking on the journey of building nutrient-rich blends is akin to sculpting a masterpiece, each ingredient, each choice, contributes to the vibrant canvas of your well-being. In this section, we will delve into the essential building blocks, unraveling the art of selecting the right fruits and vegetables, seamlessly incorporating high-protein ingredients, and achieving the delicate balance of macronutrients in your smoothies. Let's embark on this culinary adventure together, unlocking the potential of your blender to create blends that not only tantalize the taste buds but also fortify your body with the essential nutrients needed post-bariatric surgery.

Selecting the Right Fruits and Vegetables:

The foundation of any nutrient-rich blend lies in the careful selection of fruits and vegetables. Picture your blender as a palette, and each ingredient as a stroke of color contributing to a culinary masterpiece. Diverse, vibrant, and nutrient-packed, these are the qualities we seek in our ingredients.

Colorful Array of Fruits:

Envision the spectrum of colors found in fruits, from the deep purples of blueberries to the radiant oranges of mangoes. Each hue signifies a unique set of vitamins, antioxidants, and phytonutrients. Berries, rich in antioxidants, contribute a burst of flavor and immune-boosting properties. Bananas offer creaminess and a natural sweetness, while citrus fruits provide a zing of freshness.

Nutrient-Dense Vegetables:

Vegetables, the unsung heroes of nutrient density, bring a wealth of vitamins, minerals, and fiber to your blends. Leafy greens like spinach and kale introduce a verdant richness, while carrots and beets add earthy sweetness. Avocado, with its creamy texture, not only enhances the mouthfeel but also provides heart-healthy monounsaturated fats.

The key is variety. Embrace a rainbow of colors, ensuring a broad spectrum of nutrients that cater to your body's post-bariatric needs. Experiment with seasonal produce, and let your taste buds guide the way.

Incorporating High-Protein Ingredients:

Protein stands as the cornerstone of post-bariatric nutrition, facilitating healing, preserving muscle mass, and supporting sustained energy levels. Infusing your blends with high-protein ingredients transforms them into potent elixirs that nurture your body from within.

Greek Yogurt:

Creamy, rich, and teeming with protein, Greek yogurt becomes a luscious addition to your blends. It not only contributes a velvety texture but also introduces probiotics, fostering a healthy gut environment.

Nut Butters:

Elevate the protein content with the inclusion of nut butters such as almond, peanut, or cashew. Beyond their protein prowess, these butters impart a delightful nutty flavor, adding depth to your blends.

Protein Powder:

For an extra protein boost, consider incorporating high-quality protein powder.

Options range from whey to plant-based varieties, allowing you to tailor your blends to your dietary preferences.

Silken Tofu:

Silken tofu, with its neutral taste, seamlessly integrates into blends, imparting a silky texture and a protein punch. A great choice for those seeking plant-based sources of protein.

By infusing your blends with these high-protein powerhouses, you not only support your recovery journey but also transform your beverages into satisfying and nourishing treats.

Balancing Macronutrients in Your Smoothies:

Achieving the perfect balance of macronutrients – proteins, carbohydrates, and fats – is the key to crafting blends that not only taste exquisite but also provide sustained energy and satiety. Think of macronutrients as musical notes, each playing a distinct role in the harmonious composition of your smoothies.

Proteins:

The focal point of your post-bariatric blends, proteins form the backbone of your nutritional composition. Aim for a balance that aligns with your individual protein requirements, ensuring that each sip contributes to your daily protein goals.

Carbohydrates:

Carbohydrates, sourced from fruits and vegetables, provide the energy needed for your active lifestyle. The natural sugars in fruits offer sweetness, while the fiber content ensures a gradual release of energy, preventing blood sugar spikes.

Fats:

Embrace healthy fats as the supporting cast, adding richness and satiety to your blends. Avocado, nut butters, or a drizzle of flaxseed oil contribute essential fatty acids, promoting heart health and enhancing the overall mouthfeel.

Creating a well-balanced blend is a dynamic process, and personal preferences play a significant role. Experiment with ingredient ratios, listen to your body's cues, and adjust according to your taste and nutritional goals.

As you venture into the world of nutrient-rich blends, envision your blender as a magical cauldron, where the alchemy of fruits, vegetables, proteins, and macronutrients unfolds. Each blend becomes a bespoke creation, tailored to support your post-bariatric journey with flavors that invigorate your senses and nutrients that nourish your body from within. The path to vibrant wellness awaits, one sip at a time.

20 EXPERT-RECOMMENDED SMOOTHIE RECIPES

1. Morning Sunshine Protein Boost

Ingredients:

- 1/2 cup Greek yogurt

- 1/2 cup unsweetened almond milk

- 1/2 cup of frozen or fresh pineapple chunks

- 1/2 banana

- 1 scoop vanilla protein powder

Preparation:

1. Blend all ingredients until smooth. Add ice if desired.

Portion Size: 1 cup

Preparation Time: 5 minutes

Nutritional Information:

Calories: 200 | Protein: 20g | Carbohydrates: 25g | Fat: 3g | Fiber: 4g

2. Berry Blast Antioxidant Smoothie

Ingredients:

- 1/2 cup mixed berries (strawberries, blueberries, raspberries)
- 1/4 cup cottage cheese
- 1/2 cup water or unsweetened almond milk
- 1 tablespoon chia seeds
- 1 scoop unflavored protein powder

Preparation:

- Blend all ingredients until smooth. Adjust liquid for desired consistency.

Portion Size: 1 cup

Preparation Time: 5 minutes

Nutritional Information:

Calories: 180 | Protein: 22g | Carbohydrates: 15g | Fat: 5g | Fiber: 7g

Ingredients:

- 1/2 cup spinach leaves
- 1/2 cup pineapple chunks (fresh or frozen)
- 1/2 banana
- 1/4 avocado
- 1/2 cup coconut water
- 1 scoop unflavored protein powder

Preparation:

- Blend all ingredients until smooth. Add water if needed.

Portion Size: 1 cup

Preparation Time: 7 minutes

Nutritional Information:

Calories: 220 | Protein: 18g | Carbohydrates: 30g | Fat: 7g | Fiber: 6g

4. Creamy Almond Delight Shake

Ingredients:

- 1 cup unsweetened almond milk
- 1/4 cup Greek yogurt
- 1 tablespoon almond butter
- 1/2 teaspoon cinnamon
- 1 scoop vanilla protein powder

Preparation:

- Blend all ingredients until smooth. Add ice cubes for extra thickness.

Portion Size: 1 cup

Preparation Time: 5 minutes

Nutritional Information:

Calories: 220 | Protein: 23g | Carbohydrates: 12g | Fat: 10g | Fiber: 4g

5. Avocado Dream Smoothie

Ingredients:

- 1/2 avocado
- 1/2 cup spinach leaves
- 1/2 cup cucumber, peeled and chopped
- 1/2 cup unsweetened almond milk
- 1 scoop unflavored protein powder

Preparation:

- Blend all ingredients until smooth. Adjust liquid for desired consistency.

Portion Size: 1 cup

Preparation Time: 6 minutes

Nutritional Information:

Calories: 230 | Protein: 20g | Carbohydrates: 15g | Fat: 12g | Fiber: 8g

6. Chocolate Peanut Butter Paradise

Ingredients:

- 1 cup unsweetened almond milk
- 1/2 banana
- 1 tablespoon natural peanut butter
- 1 tablespoon cocoa powder
- 1 scoop chocolate protein powder

Preparation:

- Blend all ingredients until smooth. Add water if needed.

Portion Size: 1 cup

Preparation Time: 5 minutes

Nutritional Information:

Calories: 250 | Protein: 25g | Carbohydrates: 22g | Fat: 10g | Fiber: 6g

7. Pumpkin Pie Protein Delight

Ingredients:

- 1/2 cup canned pumpkin
- 1/2 banana
- 1/2 teaspoon pumpkin spice
- 1/2 cup unsweetened almond milk
- 1 scoop vanilla protein powder

Preparation:

- Blend all ingredients until smooth. Adjust spices to taste.

Portion Size: 1 cup

Preparation Time: 6 minutes

Nutritional Information:

Calories: 210 | Protein: 22g | Carbohydrates: 22g | Fat: 5g | Fiber: 7g

8. Mango Tango Cheesecake Smoothie

Ingredients:

- 1/2 cup mango chunks (fresh or frozen)
- 1/4 cup cottage cheese
- 1/2 cup water or coconut water
- 1 tablespoon chia seeds
- 1 scoop vanilla protein powder

Preparation:

- Blend all ingredients until smooth. Adjust liquid for desired consistency.

Portion Size: 1 cup

Preparation Time: 5 minutes

Nutritional Information:

Calories: 190 | Protein: 20g | Carbohydrates: 18g | Fat: 5g | Fiber: 6g

Ingredients:

- 1 cup unsweetened almond milk
- 1/2 banana
- 1 tablespoon almond butter
- 1/2 teaspoon cinnamon
- 1 scoop vanilla protein powder

Preparation:

- Blend all ingredients until smooth. Add ice cubes for extra thickness.

Portion Size: 1 cup

Preparation Time: 5 minutes

Nutritional Information:

Calories: 240 | Protein: 24g | Carbohydrates: 15g | Fat: 11g | Fiber: 5g

10. Energizing Morning Sunshine Smoothie

Ingredients:

- 1/2 cup orange juice
- 1/2 banana
- 1/2 cup Greek yogurt
- 1 tablespoon chia seeds
- 1 scoop unflavored protein powder

Preparation:

- Blend all ingredients until smooth. Adjust liquid for desired consistency.

Portion Size: 1 cup

Preparation Time: 4 minutes

Nutritional Information:

Calories: 200 | Protein: 18g | Carbohydrates: 25g | Fat: 4g | Fiber: 5g

11. Quinoa Crunch Protein Shake

Ingredients:

- 1/4 cup cooked quinoa (cooled)
- 1/2 cup mixed berries (strawberries, blueberries)
- 1/2 cup almond milk
- 1 scoop vanilla protein powder
- 1/2 teaspoon honey (optional)

Preparation:

- Blend all ingredients until smooth. Adjust sweetness with honey if desired.

Portion Size: 1 cup

Preparation Time: 6 minutes

Nutritional Information:

Calories: 220 | Protein: 22g | Carbohydrates: 25g | Fat: 4g | Fiber: 5g

12. Citrus Grilled Chicken Fusion

Ingredients:

- 1/2 cup grilled chicken breast, cooked and cooled
- 1/2 cup orange juice
- 1/4 cup Greek yogurt
- 1/2 cup water or coconut water
- 1 scoop unflavored protein powder

Preparation:

- Blend all ingredients until smooth. Adjust liquid for desired consistency.

Portion Size: 1 cup

Preparation Time: 7 minutes

Nutritional Information:

Calories: 240 | Protein: 28g | Carbohydrates: 20g | Fat: 5g | Fiber: 3g

Ingredients:

- 1/2 cup zucchini, peeled and chopped
- 1/2 cup green apple, cored and sliced
- 1/2 cup cucumber, peeled and chopped
- 1/2 cup water or coconut water
- 1 scoop unflavored protein powder

Preparation:

- Blend all ingredients until smooth. Adjust liquid for desired consistency.

Portion Size: 1 cup

Preparation Time: 6 minutes

Nutritional Information:

Calories: 190 | Protein: 20g | Carbohydrates: 25g | Fat: 3g | Fiber: 5g

14. Spicy Sweet Potato Pie Smoothie

Ingredients:

- 1/2 cup cooked sweet potato, cooled
- 1/2 banana
- 1/4 teaspoon cinnamon
- 1/4 teaspoon nutmeg
- 1/2 cup almond milk
- 1 scoop vanilla protein powder

Preparation:

- Blend all ingredients until smooth. Adjust spices to taste.

Portion Size: 1 cup

Preparation Time: 5 minutes

Nutritional Information:

Calories: 220 | Protein: 21g | Carbohydrates: 28g | Fat: 4g | Fiber: 6g

Ingredients:

- 1/4 cup feta cheese
- 1/2 cup cucumber, peeled and chopped
- 1/2 cup cherry tomatoes
- 1/4 cup Kalamata olives, pitted
- 1/2 cup water or coconut water
- 1 scoop unflavored protein powder

Preparation:

- Blend all ingredients until smooth. Adjust liquid for desired consistency.

Portion Size: 1 cup

Preparation Time: 6 minutes

Nutritional Information:

Calories: 200 | Protein: 22g | Carbohydrates: 18g | Fat: 9g | Fiber: 5g

Ingredients:

- 1/2 cup frozen cherries
- 1 cup unsweetened almond milk
- 1 tablespoon almond butter
- 1 tablespoon cocoa powder
- 1 scoop chocolate protein powder

Preparation:

- Blend all ingredients until smooth. Add water if needed.

Portion Size: 1 cup

Preparation Time: 5 minutes

Nutritional Information:

Calories: 240 | Protein: 25g | Carbohydrates: 20g | Fat: 9g | Fiber: 6g

17. Blueberry Bliss Protein Shake

Ingredients:

- 1/2 cup blueberries (fresh or frozen)
- 1/4 cup cottage cheese
- 1/2 cup almond milk
- 1 tablespoon chia seeds
- 1 scoop vanilla protein powder

Preparation:

- Blend all ingredients until smooth. Adjust liquid for desired consistency.

Portion Size: 1 cup

Preparation Time: 5 minutes

Nutritional Information:

Calories: 190 | Protein: 20g | Carbohydrates: 18g | Fat: 5g | Fiber: 7g

Ingredients:

- 1/2 cup cucumber, peeled and chopped
- 1/4 cup fresh mint leaves
- 1/2 cup green apple, cored and sliced
- 1/2 cup water or coconut water
- 1 scoop unflavored protein powder

Preparation:

- Blend all ingredients until smooth. Adjust liquid for desired consistency.

Portion Size: 1 cup

Preparation Time: 5 minutes

Nutritional Information:

180 calories, 18g of protein, 22g of carbohydrate, 3g of fat, and 6g of fibre.

Ingredients:

- 1 cup kale leaves, stems removed
- 1/2 cup of frozen or fresh pineapple chunks
- 1/2 banana
- 1/4 avocado
- 1/2 cup coconut water
- 1 scoop unflavored protein powder

Preparation:

- Blend all ingredients until smooth. Add water if needed.

Portion Size: 1 cup

Preparation Time: 7 minutes

Nutritional Information:

Calories: 220 | Protein: 20g | Carbohydrates: 30g | Fat: 7g | Fiber: 6g

20. Greek Yogurt Berry Burst

Ingredients:

- 1/2 cup Greek yogurt
- 1/2 cup mixed berries (strawberries, blueberries, raspberries)
- 1/2 cup water or coconut water
- 1 tablespoon chia seeds
- 1 scoop vanilla protein powder

Preparation:

- Blend all ingredients until smooth. Adjust liquid for desired consistency.

Portion Size: 1 cup

Preparation Time: 5 minutes

Nutritional Information:

Calories: 190 | Protein: 22g | Carbohydrates: 20g | Fat: 4g | Fiber: 7g

20 EXPERT-RECOMMENDED JUICING RECIPES

1. Green Revitalizer Juice

Ingredients:

- 1 cucumber, peeled
- 2 cups spinach leaves
- 1 green apple, cored
- 1/2 lemon, peeled
- 1-inch piece of ginger

Preparation:

- Run all ingredients through a juicer. Stir and serve over ice.

Portion Size: 1 cup

Preparation Time: 10 minutes

Nutritional Information:

Calories: 60 | Protein: 2g | Carbohydrates: 15g | Fat: 0.5g | Fiber: 3g

2. Citrus Infusion Burst

Ingredients:

- 2 oranges, peeled
- 1 grapefruit, peeled
- 1 lemon, peeled
- 1/2-inch turmeric root

Preparation:

- Juice all citrus fruits and turmeric. Mix well and enjoy immediately.

Portion Size: 1 cup

Preparation Time: 5 minutes

Nutritional Information:

Calories: 80 | Protein: 2g | Carbohydrates: 20g | Fat: 0.5g | Fiber: 4g

3. Berry Bliss Antioxidant Juice

Ingredients:

- 1 cup mixed berries (blueberries, raspberries, strawberries)
- 1/2 cup watermelon, cubed
- 1/2 cucumber, peeled
- 1/2 lime, peeled

Preparation:

- Juice all ingredients together. Serve over ice.

Portion Size: 1 cup

Preparation Time: 7 minutes

Nutritional Information:

Calories: 70 | Protein: 2g | Carbohydrates: 18g | Fat: 0.5g | Fiber: 4g

Ingredients:

- 1 cup pineapple chunks
- 1/2 apple, cored
- 1-inch piece of ginger

Preparation:

- Run pineapple, apple, and ginger through a juicer. Stir well before serving.

Portion Size: 1 cup

Preparation Time: 5 minutes

Nutritional Information:

Calories: 90 | Protein: 1g | Carbohydrates: 22g | Fat: 0.5g | Fiber: 2g

5. Carrot Orange Sunrise

Ingredients:

- 4 carrots, peeled
- 2 oranges, peeled
- 1/2 lemon, peeled

Preparation:

- Juice carrots, oranges, and lemon. Mix and serve immediately.

Portion Size: 1 cup

Preparation Time: 8 minutes

Nutritional Information:

Calories: 90 | Protein: 2g | Carbohydrates: 22g | Fat: 0.5g | Fiber: 4g

6. Red Radiance Beet Juice

Ingredients:

- 1 beet, peeled
- 1 cup strawberries, hulled
- 1/2 apple, cored
- 1/2 lemon, peeled

Preparation:

- Juice beet, strawberries, apple, and lemon. Stir well and enjoy.

Portion Size: 1 cup

Preparation Time: 7 minutes

Nutritional Information:

Calories: 80 | Protein: 2g | Carbohydrates: 20g | Fat: 0.5g | Fiber: 4g

Ingredients:

- 1 cup watermelon, cubed
- 1 cup honeydew melon, cubed
- 1/2 cucumber, peeled
- Handful of fresh mint leaves

Preparation:

- Juice watermelon, honeydew, cucumber, and mint. Serve over ice.

Portion Size: 1 cup

Preparation Time: 6 minutes

Nutritional Information:

Calories: 60 | Protein: 1g | Carbohydrates: 15g | Fat: 0.5g | Fiber: 2g

8. Kale Pineapple Zinger

Ingredients:

- 2 cups kale leaves, stems removed
- 1 cup pineapple chunks
- 1/2 apple, cored
- 1/2 lemon, peeled

Preparation:

- Run kale, pineapple, apple, and lemon through a juicer. Mix well and enjoy.

Portion Size: 1 cup

Preparation Time: 8 minutes

Nutritional Information:

Calories: 70 | Protein: 2g | Carbohydrates: 18g | Fat: 0.5g | Fiber: 3g

9. Cucumber Basil Cooler

Ingredients:

- 1 cucumber, peeled
- 1 cup fresh basil leaves
- 1 lime, peeled
- 1/2 green apple, cored

Preparation:

- Juice cucumber, basil, lime, and apple. Stir and serve over ice.

Portion Size: 1 cup

Preparation Time: 6 minutes

Nutritional Information:

Calories: 50 | Protein: 1g | Carbohydrates: 12g | Fat: 0.5g | Fiber: 3g

10. Tropical Turmeric Twist

Ingredients:

- 1 cup pineapple chunks
- 1/2 mango, peeled and cubed
- 1/2-inch turmeric root
- 1/2 lime, peeled

Preparation:

- Run pineapple, mango, turmeric, and lime through a juicer. Mix well.

Portion Size: 1 cup

Preparation Time: 7 minutes

Nutritional Information:

Calories: 80 | Protein: 1g | Carbohydrates: 20g | Fat: 0.5g | Fiber: 3g

11. Spinach Apple Ginger Boost

Ingredients:

- 2 cups spinach leaves
- 1/2 apple, cored
- 1/2-inch ginger
- 1/2 lemon, peeled

Preparation:

- Juice spinach, apple, ginger, and lemon. Stir and serve immediately.

Portion Size: 1 cup

Preparation Time: 6 minutes

Nutritional Information:

Calories: 60 | Protein: 1g | Carbohydrates: 15g | Fat: 0.5g | Fiber: 3g

12. Blueberry Basil Bliss Juice

Ingredients:

- 1 cup blueberries (fresh or frozen)
- 1/2 cup fresh basil leaves
- 1/2 cucumber, peeled
- 1/2 lime, peeled

Preparation:

- Juice blueberries, basil, cucumber, and lime. Mix well and serve over ice.

Portion Size: 1 cup

Preparation Time: 7 minutes

Nutritional Information:

Calories: 70 | Protein: 2g | Carbohydrates: 18g | Fat: 0.5g | Fiber: 4g

13. Pineapple Mint Detox Elixir

Ingredients:

- 1 cup pineapple chunks
- Handful of fresh mint leaves
- 1/2 cucumber, peeled
- 1/2 lemon, peeled

Preparation:

- Run pineapple, mint, cucumber, and lemon through a juicer. Stir well.

Portion Size: 1 cup

Preparation Time: 6 minutes

Nutritional Information:

Calories: 70 | Protein: 1g | Carbohydrates: 18g | Fat: 0.5g | Fiber: 3g

Ingredients:

- 1 cup fresh cranberries
- 2 oranges, peeled
- 1/2 apple, cored
- 1/2-inch ginger

Preparation:

- Juice cranberries, oranges, apple, and ginger. Mix and serve over ice.

Portion Size: 1 cup

Preparation Time: 8 minutes

Nutritional Information:

Calories: 80 | Protein: 2g | Carbohydrates: 20g | Fat: 0.5g | Fiber: 4g

15. Pear Ginger Zest Juice

Ingredients:

- 2 pears, cored
- 1/2-inch ginger
- 1/2 lemon, peeled

Preparation:

- Run pears, ginger, and lemon through a juicer. Stir well before serving.

Portion Size: 1 cup

Preparation Time: 6 minutes

Nutritional Information:

Calories: 70 | Protein: 1g | Carbohydrates: 18g | Fat: 0.5g | Fiber: 3g

16. Tomato Basil Garden Blend

Ingredients:

- 2 tomatoes
- Handful of fresh basil leaves
- 1/2 cucumber, peeled
- 1/2 lime, peeled

Preparation:

- Juice tomatoes, basil, cucumber, and lime. Stir and serve over ice.

Portion Size: 1 cup

Preparation Time: 7 minutes

Nutritional Information:

Calories: 50 | Protein: 2g | Carbohydrates: 12g | Fat: 0.5g | Fiber: 3g

Ingredients:

- 2 cups watermelon, cubed
- Handful of fresh mint leaves
- 1/2 lime, peeled
- 1/2 cucumber, peeled

Preparation:

- Juice watermelon, mint, lime, and cucumber. Mix and serve over ice.

Portion Size: 1 cup

Preparation Time: 6 minutes

Nutritional Information:

Calories: 60 | Protein: 1g | Carbohydrates: 15g | Fat: 0.5g | Fiber: 2g

18. Pomegranate Berry Burst

Ingredients:

- 1/2 cup pomegranate seeds
- 1 cup mixed berries (blueberries, raspberries, strawberries)
- 1/2 apple, cored
- 1/2 lemon, peeled

Preparation:

- Juice pomegranate seeds, berries, apple, and lemon. Stir well before serving.

Portion Size: 1 cup

Preparation Time: 7 minutes

Nutritional Information:

Calories: 80 | Protein: 2g | Carbohydrates: 20g | Fat: 0.5g | Fiber: 4g

19. Spinach Pear Delight

Ingredients:

- 2 cups spinach leaves
- 2 pears, cored
- 1/2 lemon, peeled
- 1/2-inch ginger

Preparation:

- Run spinach, pears, lemon, and ginger through a juicer. Mix well.

Portion Size: 1 cup

Preparation Time: 8 minutes

Nutritional Information:

Calories: 60 | Protein: 1g | Carbohydrates: 15g | Fat: 0.5g | Fiber: 3g

20. Kiwi Cucumber Quencher

Ingredients:

- 3 kiwis, peeled
- 1/2 cucumber, peeled
- 1/2 lime, peeled
- Handful of fresh mint leaves

Preparation:

- Juice kiwis, cucumber, lime, and mint. Stir and serve over ice.

Portion Size: 1 cup

Preparation Time: 7 minutes

Nutritional Information:

Calories: 70 | Protein: 1g | Carbohydrates: 18g | Fat: 0.5g | Fiber: 4g

12 EXERCISES FOR GASTRIC SLEEVE BARIATRIC PATIENTS

When it comes to exercise after gastric sleeve bariatric surgery, it's essential to focus on activities that promote overall well-being without putting excessive strain on the body. You should always get medical advice before beginning a new fitness regimen. Here are 12 recommended exercises for gastric sleeve bariatric patients:

1. Walking:

Description: A low-impact activity that can be easily modified based on fitness levels.

Recommendation: Start with short walks and gradually increase duration as tolerated.

2. Swimming:

Description: A gentle, full-body workout with minimal impact on joints.

Recommendation: Begin with water aerobics or swimming laps at a comfortable pace.

3. Cycling:

Description: Stationary or outdoor cycling provides a cardiovascular workout without excessive stress on joints.

Recommendation: Start with short sessions and gradually increase intensity.

4. Yoga:

Description: A combination of gentle movements, stretches, and relaxation techniques.

Recommendation: Choose beginner-friendly yoga poses, focusing on flexibility and balance.

5. Bodyweight Exercises:

Description: Incorporate bodyweight exercises like squats, lunges, and modified push-ups.

Recommendation: Perform exercises with proper form and start with a few repetitions.

6. Seated Exercises:

Description: Engage in seated exercises, including leg lifts, seated marches, and arm circles.

Recommendation: Ideal for individuals with mobility limitations.

7. Resistance Band Workouts:

Description: Use resistance bands for gentle strength training exercises.

Recommendation: Gradually increase resistance as strength improves.

8. Pilates:

Description: Focuses on core strength, flexibility, and overall body awareness.

Recommendation: Choose beginner-level Pilates routines to build core stability.

9. **Elliptical Training:**

Description: Low-impact exercise that combines elements of walking, running, and cycling.

Recommendation: Start with short sessions and adjust resistance as needed.

10. **Tai Chi:**

Description: An ancient Chinese martial art emphasizing slow, controlled movements.

Recommendation: Improves balance, flexibility, and relaxation.

11. **Gentle Stretching:**

Description: Include stretching exercises to enhance flexibility and reduce stiffness.

Recommendation: Focus on major muscle groups and hold each stretch for 15-30 seconds.

12. Stationary Rowing:

Description: A seated exercise that engages both upper and lower body muscles.

Recommendation: Start with a comfortable resistance level and gradually increase over time.

Remember, the key is to start slowly, listen to your body, and progress at a pace that feels comfortable. Consistency is crucial, and it's essential to choose activities that you enjoy to make exercise a sustainable part of your routine. Always consult with your healthcare team for personalized advice based on your specific health condition and recovery progress.

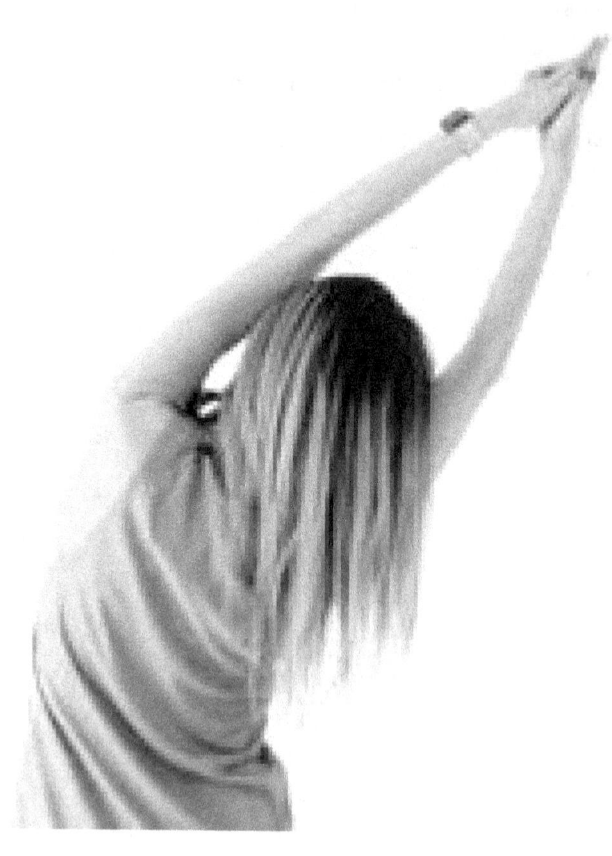

CONCLUSION

As a doctor who witnessed the positive impact of specialized recipes on my cousin sister's post-surgery recovery, I felt compelled to share this wealth of knowledge with others facing similar challenges. The success story of my previous cookbook, "Gastric Sleeve Bariatric Cookbook for Beginners," inspired me to create a dedicated resource focusing on the power of smoothies and juices.

Understanding the nuances of bariatric nutrition, the benefits of incorporating these beverages into a post-surgery diet, and the essential tools for successful blending are crucial aspects addressed in this book. By demystifying the process and presenting information in an accessible manner, my goal is to motivate and empower readers to embrace a healthy lifestyle.

Exploring the building blocks of nutrient-rich blends, including the selection of the right fruits and vegetables, incorporation of high-protein ingredients, and the delicate balance of macronutrients, serves as a fundamental guide.

This ensures not only the deliciousness of each concoction but also the fulfillment of essential nutritional requirements for a thriving recovery.

The expert-recommended 20 smoothie and 20 juicing recipes presented here are a testament to the creativity and variety that can be achieved within the confines of a post-bariatric surgery diet. Each recipe comes with detailed information on ingredients, preparation methods, portion sizes, approximate preparation times, and nutritional content. These recipes are not just nourishing but also aim to bring joy to the taste buds, making the journey towards health an enjoyable one.

In closing, I encourage readers to approach these recipes with enthusiasm, experiment with flavors, and tailor them to individual preferences. However, it's crucial to remain mindful of portion sizes and consult healthcare providers or nutritionists to ensure that these recipes align with specific dietary needs.

May this book serve as a beacon of inspiration and support, guiding individuals on a path to sustained well-being and a renewed zest for life after gastric sleeve bariatric surgery.